Handout Book for New Caregivers: Understanding and Caring for Someone with PSP

Laura Louizos

Copyright © 2024 Laura Louizos

All rights reserved.

Table of Contents

1. Understanding PSP
2. Symptoms of PSP
3. Practical Care Tips
4. Communication Strategies
5. Emotional Support and Self-Care
6. Resources and Contacts
7. Notes and Additional Details

1. Understanding PSP

What is PSP?
Progressive Supranuclear Palsy (PSP) is a rare brain disorder that affects movement, balance, vision, speech, and cognition. It results from the deterioration of cells in areas of the brain that control body movement and thinking.

Causes:
The exact cause of PSP is unknown, but it is believed to involve abnormal deposits of a protein called tau in the brain. These deposits damage nerve cells, leading to the symptoms of PSP.

Diagnosis:
Diagnosis is based on medical history, symptoms, and neurological examinations. Imaging tests like MRI can help rule out other conditions. A definitive diagnosis can be challenging and often requires consultation with a neurologist who specializes in movement disorders.

Progression:
PSP is a progressive condition, meaning symptoms worsen over time. The rate of progression can vary, but it typically advances more rapidly than other neurodegenerative diseases.

2. Symptoms of PSP

Motor Symptoms:

- **Loss of Balance and Frequent Falls:** PSP often affects balance, making falls common. This is typically one of the earliest symptoms.
- **Stiffness and Rigidity:** Muscle stiffness, particularly in the neck and upper body, is common.
- **Difficulty with Eye Movements:** Problems with moving the eyes, especially looking up and down, can cause issues with vision and balance.
- **Slurred Speech:** Changes in speech patterns, including slurring and a monotone voice, may occur.
- **Difficulty Swallowing (Dysphagia):** Swallowing difficulties can lead to choking and nutritional problems.

Cognitive and Behavioral Symptoms:

- **Slowed Thinking (Bradyphrenia):** Mental processes can slow down, making tasks that require thinking and planning more challenging.
- **Personality Changes:** Mood swings, irritability, and depression are common.

- **Apathy and Depression:** A lack of motivation and general interest in activities.
- **Difficulty with Problem-Solving and Decision-Making:** Cognitive impairments can affect daily living activities and decision-making.

Visual Symptoms:

- **Blurred or Double Vision:** Vision problems due to difficulty coordinating eye movements.
- **Sensitivity to Light:** Increased sensitivity to bright lights.
- **Difficulty Maintaining Eye Contact:** Challenges in controlling eye movements can affect social interactions.

Additional Symptoms	Notes

3. Practical Care Tips

Mobility and Safety:

- **Ensure a Safe Home Environment:** Remove tripping hazards such as loose rugs and electrical cords. Install grab bars in bathrooms and handrails on stairs.
- **Use Mobility Aids:** Walkers, canes, and wheelchairs can help prevent falls and improve mobility. Consult a physical therapist for the best options.
- **Arrange Furniture:** Keep pathways clear and arrange furniture to allow easy navigation.

Nutrition and Hydration:

- **Prepare Soft, Easy-to-Swallow Foods:** Pureed foods, soups, and smoothies can help with swallowing difficulties. Use thickening agents if necessary.
- **Encourage Small, Frequent Meals:** This can help maintain energy levels and manage swallowing difficulties. High-calorie, nutrient-dense snacks are beneficial.
- **Ensure Adequate Hydration:** Offer fluids regularly and monitor for signs of dehydration. Use a straw or adaptive cup if needed.

Communication:

- **Speak Slowly and Clearly:** Use simple sentences and repeat information if necessary. Be patient and give time for responses.
- **Use Visual Aids or Written Communication:** Pictures, flashcards, or writing on a whiteboard can help convey messages.
- **Encourage Non-Verbal Communication:** Gestures, facial expressions, and body language can be effective ways to communicate.

Daily Activities:

- **Maintain a Routine:** A structured daily routine can provide predictability and reduce anxiety.
- **Encourage Participation in Enjoyable Activities:** Engage your loved one in hobbies and activities they enjoy, adapting them as needed for their abilities.
- **Offer Assistance with Personal Care:** Help with bathing, dressing, and grooming while encouraging as much independence as possible.

4. Communication Strategies

Understanding Speech and Language Difficulties:

- **Be Aware of Speech Changes:** PSP can cause speech to become slurred or difficult to understand. Recognize these changes and adapt your communication style.
- **Use Alternative Communication Methods:** If verbal communication becomes too challenging, consider using communication boards, apps, or other assistive devices.

Engaging in Conversation:

- **Maintain Eye Contact and Be Attentive:** Show that you are listening and engaged in the conversation. This can help reduce frustration and encourage communication.
- **Use Positive Reinforcement and Encouragement:** Praise efforts to communicate, even if they are not entirely successful. Encourage attempts to express needs and feelings.
- **Allow Time for Responses:** Be patient and give your loved one the time they need to respond. Avoid interrupting or finishing sentences for them.

5. Emotional Support and Self-Care

Providing Emotional Support:

- **Listen Actively and Empathetically:** Be an attentive listener and show empathy for your loved one's feelings and experiences. Acknowledge their emotions and provide comfort.
- **Validate Feelings and Offer Reassurance:** Let your loved one know that their feelings are normal and that you are there to support them. Offer reassurance and comfort.
- **Encourage Social Interaction:** Promote participation in social activities and support groups. Connecting with others who understand their experience can provide valuable emotional support.

Self-Care for Caregivers:

- **Take Regular Breaks:** Ensure you take time for yourself to rest and recharge. Schedule regular breaks and respite care if needed.
- **Seek Support from Friends, Family, or Professional Counselors:** Don't hesitate to reach out for help. Talking to someone can provide emotional relief and practical advice.

- **Practice Stress-Reducing Activities:** Engage in activities that help you relax and reduce stress, such as meditation, exercise, or hobbies. Taking care of your own well-being is essential for providing the best care to your loved one.

6. Resources and Contacts

Support Organizations:

- **PSP Awareness:** Provides information, resources, and support for those affected by PSP. **pspawareness.com**

- **CurePSP:** Offers educational materials, support groups, and research funding for PSP and related diseases. **psp.org**

- **Local Support Groups:** Connecting with local support groups can provide a sense of community and shared experience.

Contacts

Neurologist:	
Primary Care Physician:	
Physical Therapist:	
Speech Therapist:	
Family Members:	
Nearest Hospital:	

7. Notes and Additional Details

Date	Note

Observation	Details

ABOUT THE AUTHOR

Laura Louizos is a devoted advocate and former caregiver who has dedicated herself to supporting families affected by Progressive Supranuclear Palsy (PSP) and other neurological disorders. Inspired by her personal experience caring for her mother, Coleen Cunningham, Laura founded the Coleen Cunningham Foundation to honor her mother's memory and continue her legacy of love, resilience, and unwavering strength.

For More Information and Supports Visit-
PSPAWARENESS.COM

Printed in Dunstable, United Kingdom